Kiss Me, I'm Single

an ode to
the solo life

Amanda Ford

Conari Press

First published in 2007 by Conari Press,
an imprint of Red Wheel/Weiser, LLC
With offices at:
500 Third Street, Suite 230
San Francisco, CA 94107
www.redwheelweiser.com

ISBN-10: 1-57324-301-9
ISBN-13: 978-1-57324-301-8
Library of Congress Cataloging-in-Publication Data available on request

Cover and interior design by Jessica Dacher
Typeset in August, Serifa, and Gill Sans
Cover photograph © Tatsuki Kobayashi

Printed in Canada
TCP
10 9 8 7 6 5 4 3 2 1

The paper used in this publication meets the minimum requirements of
the American National Standard for Information Sciences—Permanence of
Paper for Printed Library Materials Z39.48-1992 (R1997).

To life's wild uncertainty.

To the daring women who
embrace the unknown.

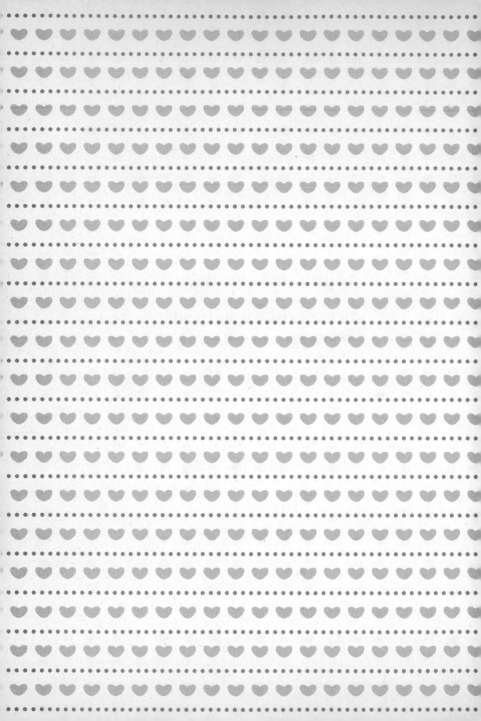

Contents

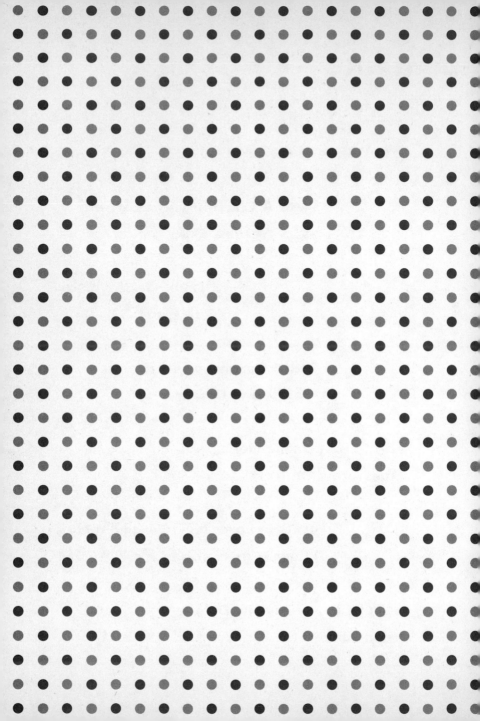

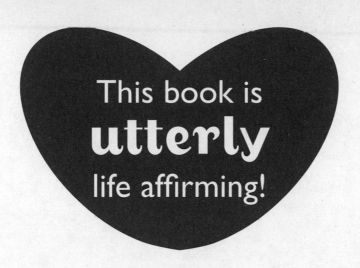

This book is **utterly** life affirming!

Amanda Ford's wisdom is urgently needed in a world where marriage is no longer the status quo.

Full of sparse prose and rousing insights, this small yet powerful book elevates singleness to new heights.

Karen Salmansohn, author of
How to be Happy, Dammit **and**
Even God Is Single

Preface

Because living alone is not easy, because the myth that love is a rare luxury enjoyed only by those in married relationships has persisted for too long, because sometimes a small book written in clear, simple, straightforward language helps more than anything, because every woman deserves to know her own beauty, deserves to discover her deepest passions, deserves to live a vibrant and joyful life regardless of her relationship status...

**I offer you *Kiss Me, I'm Single:
An Ode to the Solo Life.***

♥

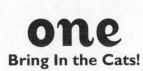

one
Bring In the Cats!

Falling in love is what happens while you are busy loving your own life.

Sometimes being a single woman feels like an emergency. It feels as urgent as Code Red when my married friends ask if I am seeing anybody special and my answer is "No" for the eighth month in a row. It feels like Code Red when my grandmother scowls and scolds, "You girls today want too much. You don't know anything about making a marriage work. You need to learn how to compromise." It feels like Code Red when I begin doing the math and figure that if I want to be pregnant by one particular age, and if I want to spend a few years traveling the world with my husband before we have children, and if I simply want to date him for a few years before we get engaged, then I should have met him **fifteen months ago.**

Fifteen months ago! **Code Red! Emergency!** We have a spinster in the making here, a young maid on the verge of becoming an old one, a lonely lady, a mistress without a man, a hag. Send her away to a rickety old shack. Bring in the cats.

It is not easy to be a single woman, and sometimes I wonder if it is even possible to be a woman without a man, because with no man a woman is just a W and an O and together those letters sound like whoa. Whoa like a horse out of control. Whoa like pulling back hard on the reigns, trying to calm her down, trying to stop her. Whoa there girl! Don't run that way. Don't buck. Don't throw your head back and holler nay. **Nay! Nope! No way! Never!** A woman without a man? Not possible.

Woe is me then, and woe is us. Woe to the women who live alone and long for love. Woe to the women who are scared of alone and so settle for men who make them only moderately happy. Woe to us with holes in our hearts that seem impossible to fill. Woe to us who are lonely by ourselves and to us who are lonely in the company of others. It is nothing but woe trying to keep bellies flat, rear ends toned, fingernails trimmed, hairs plucked, in hopes that these things will bring us some male attention. And woe is the only thing that can be said on those days when our breath comes in sighs, those days when our hearts beat prayers of longing: **Help me, help me, help me.**

Wait! Take a deep breath! Calm down! **Relax!** Don't worry! It's just a false alarm. All this talk of romantic relationships being the only place to find fulfillment in life, all this talk of love being scarce—it's Chicken Little chatter making us frantic for no reason at all.

Being a single woman is not easy,
but it is not an emergency either.
Being single is the natural state of life.
Think of it: We are each born single,
born solo, born uniquely our own
individual. Even twins enter
this world one at a time.

I am not saying that romantic relationships are an unworthy pursuit. The desire to share your life with another person is real and as natural as being born in the buff. We must search tirelessly for love. We must keep our hearts open and ready to relate, for relationships help us expand beyond the narrow confines of our own existence.

Relationships help us grow.

They help us become kinder, softer, more compassionate to the people around us. Relationships offer security and comfort and can help to quiet those existential worries that wail like banshees in our minds. These are beautiful treasures and all worth a grand quest.

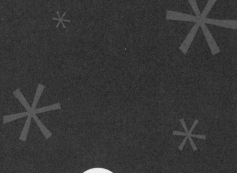

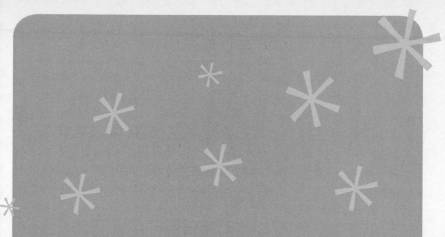

But do not be so intent on finding another that you forgot to see yourself. Do not be one of those foolish women who think that the love they give themselves is less important and less fulfilling than the love they get from men. Believe that it is just as important for you to get to know yourself as it is for you to get to know your lover. Believe that the love you offer yourself is essential and divine. Believe that the most important relationship you will ever have in your life is the one that you have with yourself. Believe it down to your bones: The search for another person must never preclude the search for yourself.

Of course,
belief alone does not
make the endeavor easy.
Love is never easy, and
self-love is the most
difficult love of all.

I have said it before
and I will say it again.
Being a single woman
is not easy.

I know a woman who wants nothing more than a husband. Every time a man crosses her path she sprints toward him with her arms jetting forward, her hands spread ready to make the grab. With each man she shouts, **"This is it. He is the one. I am in love. In love I tell you. In love!"** He never is the one, however. All the men run away. Of course they do. Nobody likes to be smothered, not even when the smothering comes backed by good intentions.

I know a woman who is waiting for a man to bring her to life. She has not cultivated a passionate interest, a deep friendship, or a fulfilling career. It seems that there is nothing to know about her except that she wants to be loved by a man. She talks incessantly about her dates and rarely about more. When I am with her I wonder if there is anything else in this wide world that brings her joy. Does she like to read? Does she listen to music? Does she take walks and notice the birds? Does she have any desires other than sex? When I imagine how she spends her time when she is home alone all I see is her sitting on the couch staring out the window with the television on in the background, waiting. This woman's relationships never last long. Although it may seem like a romantic ideal to be everything to another person, in reality such a relationship quickly reveals itself as the codependency it truly is and ends up feeling like a heavy burden for at least one person.

I know a woman who longs to love and be loved so deeply that she never utters the word. She is like a superstitious child carefully guarding her birthday wish for fear that it will never come true if she shares it with the world. Vulnerability is her enemy, and so this woman masks her anguish by smiling confidently and telling cliché jokes about the incompetence of the entire male species. If Cupid himself pulled back his bow at this very moment and penetrated her chest with an arrow, she would not feel it. **She holds herself too tightly.**

I know a woman who says she loves her boyfriend too much to let him go. She says that she cannot imagine finding another as wonderful as him. But he does not kiss her in the way she would like him to, and so she often finds herself wondering what it would be like to press her lips to those of another man. Since she will not fully commit to her boyfriend nor fully commit to leaving him, she lives in a state of limbo and says she will probably cheat. I am amazed when she tells me that she is amazed by the dissatisfaction she often feels in her relationship. What is the big surprise? Partial devotion is never fulfilling.

The time has come to put aside your commitment issues and say your vows. No more ambivalence. **No more doubting.** Pull a pair of wool socks over those cold feet. **Warm up. Jump in. Say yes.** Create an existence that is full of joy regardless of your relationship status. Vow to enter a lifelong love affair with yourself. This is the first priority.

Love has nothing to do with another person. **Love is a state of being.** It is the way in which you interact with life. Make this your mantra: Love has nothing to do with another person, but is the condition of my own heart. Say it. Mean it. Memorize it. Repeat it. Live it. Love has nothing to do with another person, but is the condition of my own heart.

My college creative writing professor often told us that in order to become successful writers we could not depend on inspiration alone. While it will certainly offer a few brilliant sentences now and again and possibly even complete a story once or twice, inspiration is much too fickle of a friend to sustain an entire career. Writing requires focused work, it requires routine, it requires commitment. Beautiful, publishable, profitable stories do not jump effortlessly onto the page the minute an author sits down to write. Great writing is crafted during weeks and months and years of careful attention.

"You must make yourself a vessel worthy of the muses to enter," my creative writing professor used to say. "Perspiration breeds inspiration." She meant we had to work first and reap the rewards second. She meant we had to write and write and write and keep writing even when we had nothing more to say. She meant that the muses are breathtaking creatures who would not be caught dead helping half-assed wannabes who spend all their time talking about becoming writers, but never actually make the commitment to sit down at their desks and write.

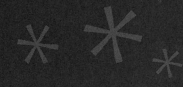

Creating a joyful life is a lot like writing. It requires the same steadfast dedication and thoughtful awareness needed to entice the muses. Fulfillment does not grace the hearts of those who laze around or complain or wallow in jealousy and self-pity. Fulfillment and joy come only to those who continually strive to know and love themselves.

Get off your derrière and get to work. Go inward and be relentless in your search. **Discover what it is that you must do to bring joy into your own life.** Educate yourself. Read about Jesus. Read about Buddha. Discover feminism and philosophy and psychology and poetry. Open up. But remember that emotional growth is not easy. You will see some ugly things lurking inside yourself, and you will have to work very hard to clean that gunk and transform it into something clear and life affirming. If you do it right, it will hurt. If you do it right you will probably cry. You will probably scream. You will probably feel like it is hopeless at times, but really it is worth it. Oh yes, Sweet Friend, the work is worth it.

two

**A Chain Is Only as
Strong as
Its Weakest Link**

It is a basic fact of life that in order to be truly happy and fulfilled with another person, you must be truly happy and fulfilled on your own first. A good relationship can enhance life for sure, but it cannot take what is only moderately satisfying and turn it into perfection.

I once lived with a man. I once wore a diamond on my left ring finger. I once had a wedding in a garden with blooming flowers, glowing bridesmaids, and a groom whose eyes filled with tears as we exchanged our vows. My eyes did not fill with tears on that day, however. Instead I cried for the entire week before our wedding. I guess this should have been the first sign that things between Evan and I were not right: Tears too early and for all the wrong reasons.

My sobs began again on the day Evan and I returned from our honeymoon and continued for the next year and half. I cried the hardest on the day that I visited a girlfriend from college at her new apartment. My friend owned a white couch that she decorated with large red and pink velvet throw pillows. I had always dreamed of owning a couch like that, but Evan detested white furnishings and turned his nose up at the combination of red and pink. On the day Evan and I went furniture shopping, I swallowed my dream and settled for beige.

I told myself it was just a couch. I said it was superficial to place so much value on the color scheme of my living room. **I reminded myself that marriage needed compromise.** I tried to convince myself that the color of the couch was not so bad, that it was a nice, neutral tone and certainly more practical than bright white. But way down, in the deepest, most secret recesses of my heart, I knew I could not spend my life sitting on beige.

I have no desire to make decisions based on practicality alone. I want to live in color. I want to live a dream. Evan saw these desires of mine as flighty, unrealistic, and utterly annoying, while I found his levelheadedness lifeless and bland. I guess it is no surprise that our marriage ended. **When a husband and wife can be nothing but negative while discussing each other's way of acting in the world, love and understanding certainly will not thrive.**

Evan and I were twenty-two when we got married, so it will probably come as no surprise to you when I say that I had not spent enough time alone fulfilling my own dreams before I became a wife. When we were engaged, women often looked at the ring on my finger and gasped, "Oh no! You are too young." I ignored them. The lure of marriage was too strong. I wanted a man and I wanted stability. Of course I did. While growing up I had neither. I was raised by a single mother with a stereotypical deadbeat dad looming in the shadows. He appeared once in a while when I was very young, but mostly he stayed hidden. This story is not unique, so again it will probably come as no surprise when I say that I married Evan partly because he was the father I never had. Evan was honest, hardworking, handsome, and dependable. When he said he would pick me up at six, he picked me up at six, and to me that was nearly everything.

Maybe one of the places we ought to look when trying to make sense of ourselves is toward our fathers. Whether they were present or absent, loving or abusive, quiet or loud, or some combination thereof, our fathers have played a role in shaping the women we are today.

The beige couch did not cause Evan and me to separate, but it was a big, heavy symbol of the fact that I was not ready to be married. Every small compromise I made felt like a death inside me. I knew that my relationship with Evan needed to end the moment I began imagining myself encouraging my own daughters not to marry young as I had. "Travel the world," I saw myself telling my girls. **"Live alone, discover yourself, date many, many men."**

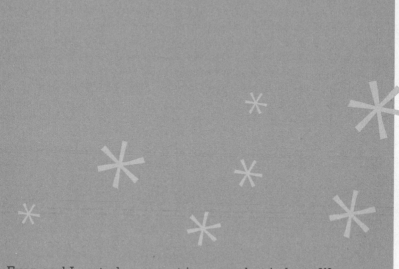

Evan and I parted ways not in anger, but in love. We knew that the relationship we had created no longer worked. **We knew that in order to grow, we had to say good-bye.** We knew that before either one of us could be part of a strong couple, we had to become strong individuals. Because isn't it true when they say that a chain is only as strong as its weakest link?

We are lucky these days. We can live for one hundred years. We can do it all. We be can be single and we can be part of a couple. In our adult lives we will most likely have a shot at both.

What good fortune! We get a shot at both. This means we must not view our single moments of life as time to search frantically for a new relationship. Enjoy your single time while you have it, because most likely it will not last forever. When it is gone you might be surprised to find yourself missing it.

My friend Erika has a boyfriend. They began dating four months ago, and that deliciously nauseating high that accompanies new love is beginning to fade as their life together stabilizes. Now they share a couple's routine. They make dinner. They cuddle on the couch. They chat on the phone. Erika, however, is missing her old routine. "I haven't written a word in weeks," she told me. "I haven't picked up my guitar, either. I spend all my time navigating the life I share with my boyfriend. I think of myself as an artist, but right now I don't feel anything like an artist. I'm in girlfriend mode and frankly I'm sort of tired of it."

My friend Georgia has a man and children whom she adores. Her husband is handsome, trustworthy, caring. The two of them prepare meals together and go dancing together. Her children often say, "I love you," and when they do it is obvious that they mean it. She has hobbies, a fit body, and a convertible to drive around the city. This woman lives a life that most women live only in their dreams. She is grateful for all of it, yet someplace deep inside her there is a sadness that she cannot articulate. She feels terrible about this. She scolds herself, she tries to stomp it down, to ignore it, but she cannot, and so Georgia wonders what to call her sadness. Is it a chemical imbalance? Is it God's punishment for a childhood transgression? Is it simply the case of a middle-class American woman who has everything and still cannot be satisfied? She is unable to figure it out, and in the end it remains with her, a longing that cannot be named.

Thus we have life with its constant longing and uncertainty. Emotional struggle is a necessary part of the human condition. Heartache is unavoidable. Individuals who are single worry. Individuals who are part of a committed relationship worry. We all worry about whether or not we are getting the most from life.

It is not easy to be a single woman, nor is it easy to be a woman in a relationship. Being a woman is not easy, and for that matter, neither is being a man. Being alive, doing your best, making the most of your time on this planet is very, very difficult.

It has been years since Evan and I separated, and if I am to be totally, completely honest, I must say that **I am so afraid of living with a man again that when I think of it, my breath stops.** I am equally scared, however, of never living with a man again, and my breath stops just the same when I imagine myself living alone from now until I die.

Fear inhabits both positions.
My mind cannot stop wondering,
"What if? What if? What if?"
What will I miss if I get married
again? What will I miss if I
remain single?

When did I start holding my breath? Was it after my divorce or long before? And what about clenching my jaw? And walking around with my shoulders so tight and so high that I can nearly wear them as earrings? When did tension become so usual, such a constant companion?

Funny that I must remind myself to breathe. Inhale and exhale. It is so natural, so essential, yet still I forget. "Take a deep breath," I coax. "Relax your jaw," I say. "Bring your shoulders down. Let go. Let go." I am working to unwind, to ease into my body, to include my breath in every moment. I am trying to remember that although I cannot see it, a divine plan for my life exists. I need not worry about the future. I cannot worry about the future. **All I can do is be present, aware of this moment, put one foot in front of the other, make one decision at a time.** Everything will fall into place in its right way and in it's right time. All I can do is trust. Down to my bones, I must trust.

three

**Getting Cozy
with Quiet**

For many women, being alone is an acquired taste. Like a fine red wine, like a potent cheese, like a rich, deep, dark chocolate, the appeal of the single life is not always apparent upon first taste.

Yesterday an acquaintance asked me, "What are you writing?" I told her that I am working on a book about creating a fulfilling life as a single woman. Upon hearing this, my acquaintance (who, by the way, is single) pursed her lips and wrinkled her nose as though she had just taken a huge bite of a lemon wedge and was expecting a sweet orange. "I would never read that," she said. "Why not?" I asked. "I don't like being single and I don't *want* to like it," she answered. "I want to be married."

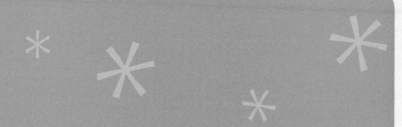

This acquaintance of mine is nowhere close to being a bride. She has no hot prospects for a groom. My acquaintance is pretty and her problem is not that men ignore her. She dates often. Instead her problem is that the men do not stick around. They leave her, I think, because she is undeveloped, a bit vapid, and shows no signs of growing into a more interesting creature. Her statement to me about not wanting to enjoy her single life is proof of the low priority she gives to personal growth.

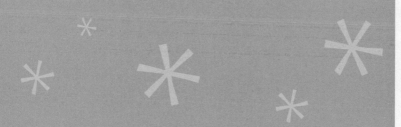

"She is an idiot," I thought to myself after I parted ways with my acquaintance. **"Doesn't she know that a man will not make her happy if she is unable to be happy by herself?** What kind of woman would make a conscious choice to not enjoy her single life? She is completely out of touch. She is out of date. Insecure! Foolish! Shallow!"

As the day went on I thought about our conversation more and my feelings toward her began to soften. I realized that what she meant by saying she did not want to like her single life was that she did not want to lose her desire to be with a man. **My acquaintance fears that if she allows herself to enjoy her single life, she might completely forget about her desire to be married and have a family.** She fears that she will become too independent, that she will become a man hater, that she will wake up on the morning of her fortieth or fiftieth or even seventieth birthday and realize that she devoted too much time to being single. My acquaintance fears that loving her single life today will lead her to loneliness in the end.

And as I thought about it even more, I realized that like my acquaintance I have a stuck place myself. **I am often so focused on building a satisfying single life that I completely ignore another desire that also resides within me: the desire to melt with a man.** I fear that if I entertain this part of myself I will become too dependent on a man and lose my identity. I worry that I will have no opinions or aspirations of my own and will become something like a wife from Stepford.

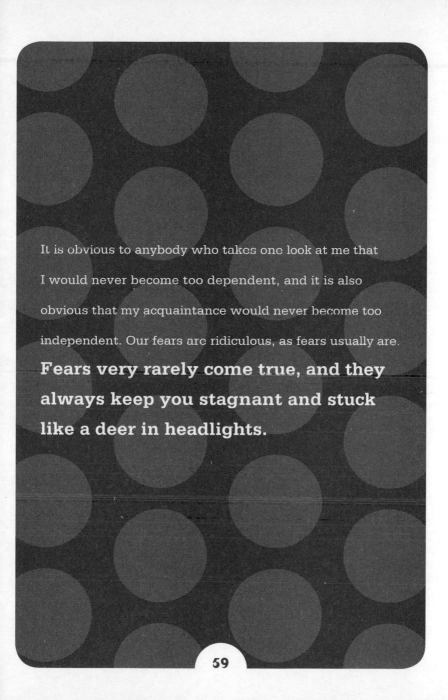

It is obvious to anybody who takes one look at me that I would never become too dependent, and it is also obvious that my acquaintance would never become too independent. Our fears are ridiculous, as fears usually are. **Fears very rarely come true, and they always keep you stagnant and stuck like a deer in headlights.**

Women who long to be married and women who long to feel satisfied on their own are not mortal enemies after all. We are not so different after all. We both have something to teach each other. It is not total dependence nor is it total independence that creates a fulfilling life, but a blend of both. A truly developed woman embraces all of her desires even when those desires seem to contradict one another. A truly developed woman examines herself with honesty and is open to what she sees. **A truly developed woman is not afraid.**

The key to loving your single life is not denying your desire for a relationship.

They key to loving your single life is being comfortable with the grey. It is remembering that life is a constant paradox. We want to find ourselves, to be comfortable standing on our own, *and* we want to lose ourselves in romance. We want to experience the excitement and possibility of the single life *and*. we want the routine and stability of a committed relationship. Life is never one or the other, but always both. Everything jumbled together happening all at once, that is truth.

So how does a woman
acquire a taste for being
alone? A woman acquires
a taste for being alone
by being alone.

And why would a woman want
to acquire a taste for being alone?
A woman wants to acquire a taste
for being alone because being
alone is sacred ground.

I am campaigning for quiet. **It's time for quiet. Vote silence! Go nothingness! Choose boring! Press mute!** Turn off your television. Turn off your cell phone. Turn off your computer. Go for a walk without your headphones. Drive your car without listening to the radio. Drink a cup of coffee without reading the paper. **It is time to sit and stare into space.** It is time to say to yourself, "Hello, Self. How are you?"

Maybe it sounds like a stupid self-esteem exercise that a New Age preschool teacher would do with her students. Hi, Self. How are you, Self? I love you, Self. I guess it is stupid in a way. **It is stupid that we are so consumed by the external world that we are completely oblivious to the internal universe.** It is stupid that people talk on cell phones in restaurants and bookstores and art galleries. It is stupid that there are entire industries dedicated to chronicling the mundane moments in the lives of celebrities. It is stupid that my friend talks about the characters of her favorite television show as though they are real people, as though they are her actual friends. It is stupid that last week when I had a seemingly unbearable moment of anxiety I rushed to the nearest clothing boutique and spent money I do not have on things I do not need or, for that matter, even want.

It is stupid that we are so disconnected from ourselves that as adults we must revert to the remedial beginnings.

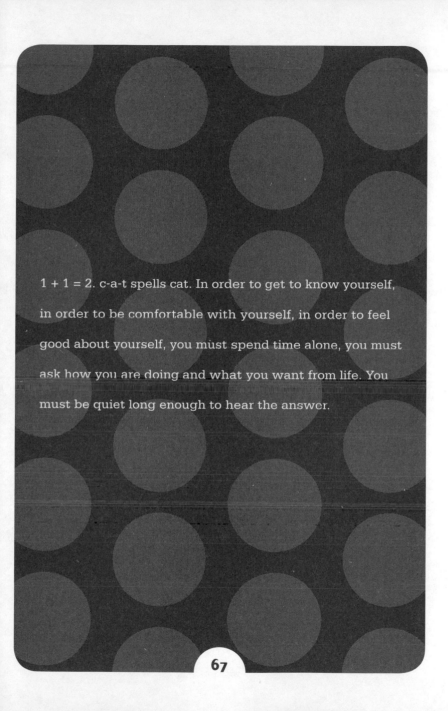

1 + 1 = 2. c-a-t spells cat. In order to get to know yourself, in order to be comfortable with yourself, in order to feel good about yourself, you must spend time alone, you must ask how you are doing and what you want from life. You must be quiet long enough to hear the answer.

I know a husband and wife who say that they are incredibly in love. They also say, however, that they both work too much and do not get to spend enough time together. To remedy this, they decided to escape to the coast for a weekend where, free from distraction, they could devote themselves to each other. They quickly discovered that the pace of that seaside town was a lot slower than they were accustomed to, and within hours the couple found that they were anxious and bored. "There was nothing to do," the husband complained as he told me about their weekend. "Yeah," the wife added, "I mean, we walked on the beach and ate clam chowder, but after that it was like, 'Now what?'" The next vacation this couple took was to Las Vegas where they had a great time, as the wife put it, "being surrounded and constantly over stimulated."

Can you even imagine?

Don't lovers want to be distracted *by* and not *from* each other? Isn't the crashing of waves background music enough for a romantic rendezvous? Who would want to be so uncomfortable with stillness that the prospect of spending just two short days staring into the eyes of her love seems boring and worthless?

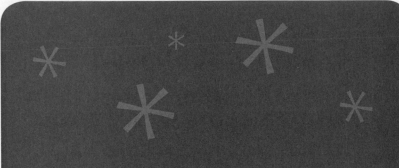

Learning to be comfortable with being alone and all the silence associated with it not only allows you to know yourself, but it **allows you to be available to those around you.** Developing a relationship with quiet makes you a better listener, a better lover, a better friend, a better daughter, a better mother, a better woman.

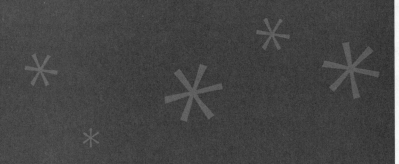

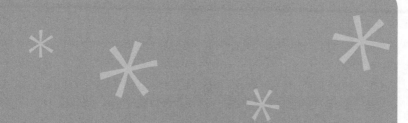

Why are we so afraid to turn off our cell phones? Why do we insist on watching television? Why can we earn advance degrees, run businesses, and give birth while barely batting an eyelash, yet the mere thought of spending a Saturday night alone makes us panic? **We are so strong, yet so weak.** We are so brave, yet so afraid.

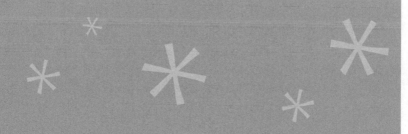

Thus we must be tender. We are vulnerable and so sweet. Yes, Dear Friend, you too. Be tender to yourself, for you are vulnerable and so sweet.

Being single is not easy.

Being alone is not easy.

Being alone is humiliating.

Being alone will bring

you to your knees.

I know a woman who has dated one guy after another after another after another since age fourteen. Now she is in her early thirties and has not spent more than, literally, two weeks being single. When one relationship ends, she finds another immediately. Sometimes she finds another relationship before her first one is officially over. This woman uses the excitement of new romance to numb the pain of dying love, but because she does not fully mourn the loss of her old boyfriends, she is unable to fully celebrate the arrival of the new ones. **To be truly grateful for a love gained, a woman must experience the pain of a love lost.**

In Seattle, where I live, the weather is mostly grey and rainy. We spend over half the year under gloomy clouds and go for weeks—weeks and weeks—without seeing even a glimpse of sun. But let me tell you, it is worth it, because the summers here are the most incredible on the planet. The hills and trees are green from months of precipitation, and the sun, oh the sun! I cannot tell you how amazing it is to feel the warmth of the sun after so long without it. True Seattleites would never trade the grey, for they know that if the sun shines year-round it loses much of its splendor. It is sort of the same with love. True romantics would never opt out of feeling the pain of a broken heart, for they know that it is this pain that helps make the joy of the next love even more vibrant.

Anxiety and fear are natural elements of life that cannot be eliminated with the latest technology, a closet full of designer clothes, a calendar booked with dinner dates, or even a husband. We can certainly use these things like a drug to numb our fear and anxiety, but to be honest, I am not sure that intentional numbing is a good option to choose. Somewhere along the line in our social evolution we began labeling any emotion that is difficult to sit with as bad. But an emotion cannot be bad, for each plays an important role in our development. While they may be extremely uncomfortable, intense sadness after a loss, anger when love is betrayed, fear at the prospect of spending a lifetime alone, free-floating anxiety that looms within us for no particular reason are natural and healthy. Allow yourself to experience these emotions. Welcome them. Do not be afraid, for they will not stay forever. Once you have given these emotions their due attention they will pack up and move on.

I do not know why it is, I just know that it is: The lower depths you descend, the higher peaks you climb. If you continually choose numb as your method for dealing with pain, you will begin to numb your joy as well, until eventually an even, numb buzz becomes your constant state of being. Numb is a deadened way to live.

There is a gravel trail around the perimeter of the small, manmade lake that sits just blocks from my apartment. That three-mile trail is a haven for runners, and when I first moved to the city, I longed to join all the people who circled the lake after work for their evening exercise. The problem was that I did not like to run. I found it uncomfortable and exhausting. The first few times I ran the lake my lungs heaved, my mind wandered, I got bored, I got tired, and I always stopped to walk long before I had completed my loop. I kept running not because I liked the act of running, I kept going because I liked the idea of being a runner. It has been four years since my first strides around the lake. Today not only is running that gravel trail easy, but it is joyful. I like to run. It is my release. It is my activity. I cannot imagine my life without it.

You may like the idea of being a self-aware, confident, open, stable woman, but unfortunately liking the idea of being this woman is not enough to make you this woman. Desire is the best motivation for sure, but still you must work, and the work you need to do in order to feel comfortable on your own is like walking barefoot across burning coals. You most likely will hate the process, but after you work through all your anxiety and fear and sadness about being single, you might find that you actually enjoy going out to dinner by yourself or that a silent Saturday night at home alone is a welcome retreat from the world of noisy stimulation and social interaction.

four

Gazpacho with Crème Fraîche and Gratitude

To nourish your body with healthy food and exercise, to control your finances by paying off debt, living within your means and saving a bit of cash each month, to use kind words when discussing your character, to forgive yourself again and again and again for all your human mistakes—these are high acts of self-love.

What more can we do in life but love ourselves? We can

have exciting careers, we can wear designer clothes, we

can get manicures and pedicures, we can go to parties

and drink martinis every Friday night. We can discuss art

and politics. We can read great literature. We can travel

the globe. All these things, however, are nothing if we do

not love ourselves. Self-love is the only thing that matters.

Without self-confidence, no true
accomplishment is possible.
If you do not love yourself, you
will never find joy in anything.
You will always be lacking.

I have a part-time job at an athletic club. Across the street is a deli where I often go for a sandwich and a cookie. While on my lunch break there one afternoon, the boy working behind the counter (he was about seventeen, maybe eighteen, years old), asked, "Don't you work at that gym?" I nodded. I am not usually excited to talk about this job. "Are you a personal trainer?" he asked. I shook my head, "No." The boy persisted, "So what do you do there?" he asked. "I just work at the front desk," I told him. He said, **"That's cool, but you shouldn't say it like that. You make your job sound so worthless."** And he was right—so young yet so wise. I had been sheepish and reluctant in my tone of voice, in my choice of words, in my body language. That boy called me out. He made me see.

Somewhere along the line I got into a bad habit of belittling my own existence. When somebody inquires about where I work, I answer, "Just at the gym." When I go for a run and a friend asks how far I went, I say, "Just three miles." When people are curious about my writing and want to know what I am working on, I tell them, "Nothing exciting. Just this little book." *Just, only, not much, boring, barely*—I am going to stop using these words to describe my life.

My friend Marla is an actress. If she could she would spend all her time on stage, but of course there are bills to pay, and so she works, as stereotype would have it, as a waitress at a trendy restaurant in Manhattan. Marla longs for the day when she no longer has to wait tables and is making her entire living by landing roles in productions on Broadway. I can relate. I want to quit my job at the gym. I want to support myself with writing alone. The last time Marla and I spoke on the phone, we complained about our situations. "I hate the restaurant," Marla said. "I hate the gym," I said. Marla told me a story about a mediocre female actor who landed a highly coveted lead role only because the director is her boyfriend's brother. I told Marla a story about an acquaintance of mine who is going back to school to become a fashion designer, only she does not have to work or take out a single loan because she has a trust fund and her father is paying her tuition.

Marla and I are endlessly jealous of women who are more successful than we are. During our last conversation, Marla told me that she actually had a daydream about sabotaging her roommate's audition when the two of them were going for the same part, and I admitted that I cannot read anything—not a book, not a magazine article, not a blog—without comparing myself to the author and tying my heart into knots with envy. It seems that everywhere Marla and I look we see somebody who is smarter, who is more talented, who works harder, who has more connections, **who is just totally, randomly, unfairly, completely luckier than we could ever imagine ourselves to be.** It is unfair. It is horrible. When will we be there? It feels like never. We are down. We are depressed. We might as well lie in the gutter. We might as well give up. We might as well die.

Sometimes it feels like no matter how hard I work, I cannot get ahead. Marla feels this too. There is no telling if she and I will ever make it, and if we do it is questionable whether or not that success will quench our thirst. Just look at us now. Both Marla and I each earn a portion of our living by doing what we love, but still we complain and want more. We are both so anxious to get on to the next thing that we refuse to enjoy today and be proud of the accomplishments we have made. I am not sure what makes Marla and me believe that we will ever be satisfied. If we cannot relax here where we are, what makes us think we will relax once we reach that elusive "there"? Won't we always find more work to do, more money to make, more recognition to gain?

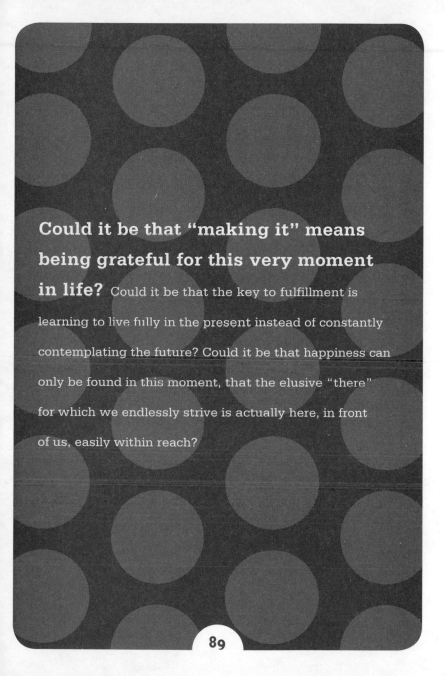

Could it be that "making it" means being grateful for this very moment in life? Could it be that the key to fulfillment is learning to live fully in the present instead of constantly contemplating the future? Could it be that happiness can only be found in this moment, that the elusive "there" for which we endlessly strive is actually here, in front of us, easily within reach?

When a woman is longing, it seems that everywhere she looks she sees a dozen other women who have the exact thing she wants. What many single women want are men. If this is the case for you, if you believe couples surround you, if you feel like there are so many women in happy, committed relationships, I must tell you that you are right. Couples do surround you. There are so many women in happy, committed relationships. In fact at this very moment there is probably a beautiful woman wrapped in a tender embrace with her doting, devoted husband. She has exactly what you want. So I must ask this question not only to you Dear Reader, Sweet Friend, but I must ask it to myself as well: What are you going to do about it? What are you going to do knowing that there are women all across the globe who posses the very thing for which you cannot stop wishing? Are you going to lie in the gutter, give up, and die?

What if God, or the fates, or a gypsy fortune-teller, or whomever it is you would trust in delivering accurate information regarding your future, came to you this very moment and told you that you will be single for the rest of your life? What would you do knowing that from now until your death you must be your own source of love, tenderness, romance, and affection? **How would you live differently?** What would you do to change your perspective?

Let me clarify that I propose the previous "what if" statement to you only because it is a good exercise to use when examining your single life. I, under no circumstances, believe that a woman who remains committed to growth and keeps her heart open will be left to be the sole provider of her own emotional support. Love is abundant. If love is what you want and if you work diligently to cultivate it, you will have it. Be forewarned, however, that it may not come in the form of Prince Charming and a white picket fence, which is fine, of course, because we all know by now that fairy tales are fiction.

I am single and I love my single life, but **I also love love.** Like I said before, truth is always *both*; it is every feeling and thought acting together all at once. As living creatures we are large and complex. We hold the universe within our souls. I am a confident single and also a hopeless romantic. I am always falling in love. I love a broken heart. I hope I still get crushes when I am eighty.

We have become quite demanding. We want romance. We want entertainment. We want diamonds on our fingers. We want mind-blowing sex. We want huge wardrobes. We want fancy vacations. We want faces without laugh lines. When we do not get these things we feel very inadequate and we get mad. Do you remember Veruca Salt from *Charlie and the Chocolate Factory*? Remember her demand, "I want an Oompa-Loompa now!" Be honest. You have acted that way before. You have thrown a tantrum: "I want new clothes. I want better friends. I want love. **I want it now. Now! Now! Now! Now!**"

I thought of something the other day that helped lighten me a little, and maybe it will help lighten you as well. We are not owed anything in life. This existence itself is a gift and for it we are forever in debt. The only way to pay back this debt is with gratitude. **Life owes me nothing, but I owe everything to life.**

It is your choice whether to view the proverbial glass of life as half-empty or half-full. You can be a Pollyanna or a Wicked Witch. You can choose to label your life as lacking and dissatisfying, or you can label it complete and fulfilling.

The good news is, our points-of-view are not set in stone, and sometimes the only thing needed to transform a so-so life into something spectacular is a change of perspective.

Maybe you are rolling your eyes right now. Maybe you think I am oversimplifying the situation. "Love yourself," I proclaim. "Change your perspective! It's a cinch! Your life will be grand! Perfect! Dazzling!" You are shaking your head. You have heard it all before. You know that what I am suggesting is much easier said than done.

You are correct, and because
you are correct, I offer you
this one, very practical, fail-
proof technique for shifting
your outlook on life:
Cook dinner for yourself.

My single friends often complain about cooking. "Cooking for one is no fun," they grumble. "It is much better to make dinner when I have somebody to eat with me." I can accept these statements as true. I cannot, however, accept them as valid reasons for a woman to give up cooking for herself altogether, because it is also a lot better to work when you earn over $100,000 a year, but does this mean a woman should refuse to take a job until she is guaranteed this salary?

Let us stop waiting for perfect circumstances. **Let us live now.** Let us be vibrant and dynamic. Let us run to the market in droves and fill our baskets with our favorite foods. Let us pull out our utensils. Let us put on ruffled aprons. Let us open a bottle of wine. Let us chop and stir and sauté and boil and bake. Let there be candles at our tables and music filling our rooms. Let our senses ignite. Let us relax and savor. Let the food be as fresh and as flavorful as us glorious, succulent, wise, single women.

Just because you are not dining with Prince Charming doesn't mean you needn't eat like a queen. Just because there is no man in your bed doesn't mean you shouldn't sleep in lacy lingerie. Just because you have not had sex in months doesn't mean you can't read the *Kama Sutra*. Hot nights are not reserved for relationships.

We are women, we are feminine, we are lovely, and we deserve to know it and show it. May we always see our beauty, whether we have men or not.

I know a single woman who loves to cook. She makes almost everything from scratch: nutty vinaigrettes, crispy, candied pecans, and pesto with fresh mint and garlic. Her specialties include a blue cheese soufflé, gazpacho with crème fraîche, spinach-stuffed veal breasts, and a lemon tart with the zest of ten lemons and a very buttery crust. She often prepares meals for her dates and after relishing her creations, with their bellies satisfied and warm, the men usually ask something like, "Will you marry me?" (Proof that the path to a man's heart truly is through his stomach.) My friend always responds, "Why get married when you can be single?"

And she means it, too. **My friend prefers to be single, and not because she isn't open to love.** Her life is full of love and romance, of deep friendships and intimate connections. It's not that she's selfish or fickle or reclusive or boring. It's just that she prefers silence over small talk, unexpected whimsy over day-to-day routine. She prefers to save her money the way she pleases and spend it when she pleases. She prefers to take a bath and practice yoga before bed. She prefers to wake up alone in the morning so that she can quietly prepare her jasmine tea and venture to the front porch to pet the neighbor's cat while he twists around her ankles.

When I say, **"Cook for yourself,"**
I do not mean open a box and stick a plastic container of
frozen food into the microwave. I mean open a cookbook
and find a recipe that excites your taste buds. Your meal
need not be complicated, but it must be fresh. Grilled fish,
roasted organic vegetables, green salad with olive oil and
toasted almonds, crème brûlée.

Food creates energy and healthy food creates healthy energy. Food is sustenance. Give great attention to what goes into your body for it is what fuels your very existence. Be aware. Learn to listen to your body, to your stomach, to your cells. **Healthy food is a basic building block.** Without it, you cannot support the life of your dreams.

If you can conquer the kitchen, if you can sit at the table for thirty minutes slowly enjoying your meal, if you can satisfy your own hunger, then you can do anything. The world is your oyster.

If you take time to educate yourself about wholesome nutrition, and make time to prepare nourishing meals and snacks, then you need not fear a thing. You have proven that you can care for yourself at the most basic, fundamental level. If you keep it up, this self-care will overflow from your plate and infuse the rest of your life.

Let loneliness erupt! Let sadness arise! Let disappointment intrude! These feelings will not devastate you. Oh no! You have the skills to soothe your own heart.

Claire never planned on being single so far into her adult life. "I'm in my forties, for crying out loud," she says. "I thought I'd be married by now. I thought I'd have teenage children." But for reasons that are impossible to pinpoint, Claire has not yet had a chance to walk that path, and if you ask her, she will tell you quite candidly that driving the single road used to make her very, very bitter. "Especially on Valentine's Day," Claire says, "with its ridiculous rose-hued romance." What a nuisance, that cheesy, smug, stupid, sentimental, saccharine, mass-marketed Hallmark holiday!

Claire felt truly awful on Valentine's Day. Out of sorts.

Dissatisfied. Lost. Unloved. Ugly. Tired. Lonely. Depressed.

It was a miserable occasion, a glaring red reminder of her

unanswered prayer for a man and a family of their own.

Claire found herself questioning God and concluding that

if a great creator did in fact exist, he was obviously

sarcastic, malevolent, and incredibly unforgiving to leave

her unmarried year after year. Claire thought God was an

idiot. "I mean, who would give a blindfolded, flying baby

a bow and arrow and let him be in charge of something so -

important as love and romance?" Damn Cupid!

But in her fortieth year of life, on the day before Valentine's Day, Claire had a moment of clarity in the least likely of places: on the couch in front of her television. "I was watching some show and the main character was this annoying single woman who spent twenty minutes criticizing the Valentine's Day plans of her coupled friends and coworkers. Right then it hit me hard: I was that woman. I had become a stupid, Friday night sitcom—a cliché." And what Claire hated even more than Valentine's Day, were stupid, Friday night sitcom clichés.

Immediately Claire fell to her knees. She begged for forgiveness. She saw the light. Valentine's Day was not her problem. *She* was her problem. "I realized that I didn't have to believe all that crap about myself. I had had some beautiful relationships in the past and just because they hadn't taken me to the altar didn't mean I had to wallow and whine on Valentine's Day." Claire turned off her television. She went to the grocery store. She bought herself a dozen red roses and a dozen pink roses and box of very fine heart-shaped chocolates. The next day— Saturday, February 14—she invited her seventy-three-year-old widowed neighbor for a dinner of seafood bisque and raspberry martinis. Claire lit candles and put on French music. Together the two women sat amongst the roses and discussed first kisses, broken hearts, and their hopes for the wild, uncertain future.

Now instead of feeling left out on Valentine's Day, Claire goes all out.

Her new attitude has reached beyond this once-hated holiday and has taken hold of the rest of her days as well. **Claire understands that love and excitement for life are things that a person develops inside;** they are not gifts randomly bestowed by a careless supernatural power. Thus Claire has softened. She is empowered. She knows that if she can provide herself with a warm and uplifting Valentine's Day, then she can do anything.

five

**Love, Unlike Money,
Does Grow on Trees**

Why is it that the
only relationships we readily
celebrate are those that lead
toward marriage? Why do we
believe that the only love worth
searching for is a romantic love
that lasts for eternity?

Have you ever ridden a bicycle at night through barren city streets? If you haven't, you must. You absolutely must!

I did it last night with my new friend, Nathan. I called him early yesterday afternoon and asked, "Do you want to see a movie tonight?" He said yes and asked, "Should we ride our bikes?" I said yes. It was nearly nine when we began pedaling to the theater and immediately I fell in love: in love with the cool air, in love with the quiet of the streets, in love with the gleaming smile of the crescent moon, in love with the fog beginning to settle, in love with my spinning legs, in love with the large cowlick in the back of Nathan's head where his hairline meets his neck.

Nathan and I met just three weeks ago and, although we connect in that indescribable way as though we know each other much better than we actually do, Nathan and I are technically "just friends." We do not kiss or hold hands or date in the traditional sense of the word. I'm not sure if I even want that with him or if he even wants that with me. I am sure, though, that last week Nathan brought me a pomegranate for no particular reason other than it is currently winter and pomegranates are in season. I guess he must have thought of me when he saw it. His gesture touched me. I ate the fruit with my breakfast the next morning and smiled. I am also sure that last night in the theater I had a deep urge to rest my head on his shoulder as we watched the film.

I am trying out a new technique with Nathan: enjoy our moments together without letting my mind kidnap those moments and run into the future. I am trying not to think about a kiss at the end of the night and trying not to predict if he will be the father of my children someday. I am trying to be comfortable with the fact that I do not have an obvious answer to the question, "What's going on with you and Nathan?" I am trying to focus on what matters, and what matters right now are juicy pomegranate seeds and jumping on bicycles on a Tuesday night in December and riding through the fog to see a movie. Who cares that there is no one word to easily describe our relationship? Who cares that it is unclear whether or not we are headed toward romance? Isn't the crisp night air against our cheeks and the smooth connection between us cause enough for celebration?

Why do we value labels so much? What do labels mean anyway? Think of it: there are married people who lie, cheat, and treat their spouses callously. The titles "husband" and "wife" have not delivered them from dishonesty and self-obsession. In truth, the label you assign to a person is minor in comparison to how you treat that person and how that person treats you. *Husband, wife, fiancé, lover, friend, acquaintance, stranger, enemy*—these are tiny words, just sounds from the mouth, incapable of expressing the complexity of human relationships.

A simple hug can convey more affection, more sympathy, more comfort, more excitement than a sentence, a paragraph, or an entire novel of words ever could. Today let us put our energies into loving the people in our lives instead of trying to fit them into tidy categories. **Today let us celebrate. Let us enjoy. Let us bask. Let us stop analyzing. Let us stop labeling.** Let us stop worrying so much about how to describe the world around us and, for one day, let us soak in life's mystical, mysterious beauty.

How does one soak up life's mystical, mysterious beauty? Good question. I'm glad you asked. **Living quietly and joyfully in the moment** is not an easy undertaking. I struggle with it daily. This type of living requires a shift from the mind to the heart, a surrendering of worry to faith, a move from the frantic world of desire and ambition to the tranquil heavens of fulfillment and thanks.

Today, ask your mind to be quiet. Ask it not to pine for the past or plan for the future. Ask for a reprieve from analyzing and classifying. Say to your mind, "Sweet Mind, relax, don't worry, fear not, all is well. I would like a reprieve. I will call on you again when there are bills to pay, meetings to attend, and work to be done, but for today I would like simply to enjoy my life, to experience living without your constant commentary."

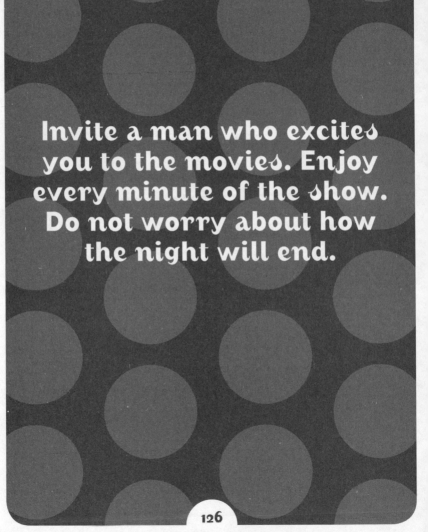

Invite a man who excites you to the movies. Enjoy every minute of the show. Do not worry about how the night will end.

If you wish to entangle your fingers with his, do. If you desire to rest your head on his shoulder, do. If you long to press your forearm against his forearm as they both sit on your shared armrest, do. Do not worry, "What is he thinking? Is this appropriate? What does it all mean?" This is not to be taken so seriously. It's just a movie. It's just love and romance, after all.

Love is not like money. It is not something to be saved and invested and spent only after careful consideration. Love *does* grow on trees. You have plenty for everybody. There is no need to hold your love tightly, no need to save it for a rainy day.

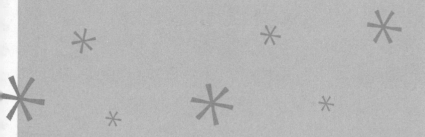

One of the gifts of singlehood is that we get to sample countless varieties of love. Because we don't have one partner to rely on for affection and support, we must instead develop a network of partners to call upon to fulfill our emotional needs. Every woman needs somebody to flirt with, somebody to vent to, somebody who makes her laugh, somebody to pick her up when her car breaks down on the side of the road, somebody to hug her when she cries and rub her head and assure her quietly,

"Everything is going to be okay."

Maybe the thought of depending upon a multitude of people feels more like a burden than a gift. After all, having a partner means you can go to the same person when you are frustrated, nervous, excited, or joyful. When you have a partner, it is obvious whom you call on for a dinner date or a ride to the dentist or sex or money or advice. It's obvious and it's easy. But in case you have not yet noticed, let me tell you: There is no such thing as one size fits all. While developing different friendships to fill your different needs certainly takes effort at first, in the end you will be better off having had intimate connections with an array of personalities. You may even find, when it's all said and done, that you turn out to be a more developed, complex, interesting individual than all those women who have been relying on the same men for everything year after year.

Instead of drinking Merlot every night, we singles can drink Merlot today and Zinfandel tomorrow. We can drink a Pinot, a Syrah, a Sangiovese, a Chardonnay, a Riesling. We can have port and grappa and Champagne. We can even have a shot of tequila and chase it with a margarita or we can spend the afternoon sipping lemonade on the porch swing out front. **Think of how refined and satisfied our palates will be having tasted all the flavors that life has to offer.**

I once read an article in a popular psychology magazine that modern-day singles have better relationship skills than their coupled counterparts. Why? Because without one person to go to for all their emotional support, singles place a high value on friendship, developing deep bonds with an array of personalities. Couples tend to put friendships on the back burner, reserving closeness only for their significant others. For couples, friendships are an accessory; for singles friendships are a necessity.

My friend Scarlett has a friend Ian. Every Tuesday Scarlett buys two slices of cake from her favorite bakery and takes them over to Ian's house. Ian makes tea, and the two sit at his kitchen counter indulging in sweets and sharing the events of their weeks. Later Ian turns on his stereo and sits at the end of the couch where Scarlett has already made herself comfortable lying with a blanket. Ian takes her feet into his lap and massages them deeply while they both lose their minds in the music. About forty minutes later, Ian walks Scarlett to her car, where they hug tightly and say, "Thank you," and, "Good night," and, **"See you next Tuesday."**

My friend Scarlett also has a friend Matthew. They met last July at the thirty-second birthday party for a shared acquaintance. The two bonded quickly, both having filled their keg cups with ice water instead of beer and showing more interest in the lovely garden blooming next door than in the fraternity-party antics booming inside. At the end of the night Scarlett and Matthew parted ways, figuring this first meeting would be their last. Matthew lived in Arizona and was only visiting Scarlett's Washington State for business. But when Matthew returned to Tucson and couldn't stop thinking of Scarlett, he found her mailing address and sent her a card telling how he enjoyed their conversation. Scarlett returned the gesture. Then Matthew wrote again. Now it is almost one year later, and while they have not met face-to-face another time, Scarlett and Matthew have cultivated a unique friendship in handwritten letters delivered by the postman three to five times each month.

My friend Scarlett calls her friend Jackie when she feels like being wild. Jackie drives a magenta Harley-Davidson and owns a hipster bar in an artsy part of town. On Saturday nights, Jackie stars in a burlesque revival, wearing four-inch high heels and a sequin bustier while chewing bubble gum and twirling a red hula hoop around her hips. Scarlett's outings with Jackie are unpredictable, thrilling, and occasionally a little bit unnerving. Thanks to Jackie, Scarlett once found herself at the top of a Ferris Wheel lip-locked with the very cute drummer of a very unknown rock band. With Jackie, Scarlett has danced on bar tops, been arrested for skinny-dipping, and even won $2,000 while playing blackjack on a spontaneous trip to Vegas.

My friend Scarlett spends a lot of time with her friend Tina. They run errands together, dine at trendy new restaurants together, and call each other just to chat. Scarlett and Tina meet for coffee, consult about clothing, haircuts, eye makeup, and exercise. They lend each other money when finances are tough and encourage each other to remain optimistic when life feels like nothing but worry and stress. Scarlett and Tina paint each other's living room walls, go for hikes, exchange gifts, watch television, recommend books, tell jokes, and even argue from time to time. To Scarlett, Tina seems like a sister, and with her Scarlett feels relaxed and natural with no reason to censor her words or calculate her actions.

My friend Scarlett visits her grandfather whenever she has time. He lives alone in a mountain bungalow ninety minutes outside of the city. When Scarlett drives to see him she brings along frozen pizza and Jell-O salad. They eat dinner while playing cards (it was from him that she learned blackjack as a young girl) and sipping scotch. Her grandfather doesn't talk much, but when she leaves he hands her a $50 bill and says, "See ya, kiddo." When Scarlett says, **"I love you,"** he nods in response and waves good-bye with a single flap of his hand.

I once asked Scarlett if she wants to get married and she answered that yes, she would very much like to have a husband. "But only if it's right," she said. "Only if it's really, really right." Scarlett does not believe that one person could fill her every need. She believes that **true spiritual, emotional, and intellectual growth come only by developing intimate connections** with a wide array of people. "My friends all take me to different places inside myself, places I would never visit if each of them weren't there to guide me."

So while Scarlett hopes to experience the type of intimacy that develops from a for-better-or-worse, day-to-day-grind, share-a-bathroom-and-a-bed sort of commitment, she doesn't want it at the expense of the other kinds of intimacy that fill her life. "I never want to be singularly focused on one person," Scarlett says. "I like spreading my time around and **sharing love with many different people.** I like being complicated."

I understand what Scarlett means. When I was married, I spent the vast majority of my free time with Evan, while occasionally squeezing engagements with friends into tiny, partitioned segments that appeared on my calendar. If you had asked me about it at the time, I would have insisted that I valued my friendships immensely. Judging by the way I focused my energies, however, it was obvious that the only relationship of true importance to me was the one with my husband. I poured everything into Evan. I made him my sole love object, my playmate, my entertainer, my shopping partner, my career advisor, my workout motivator, my family counselor, my passion igniter, my tear dryer, and my dream holder. I believed it was necessary for me to invest everything in Evan, because I had been told from a very young age that the only place a woman could find a fulfilling connection and deep bond was inside a monogamous, romantic relationship with a man.

Now that I have been single for years and have been forced to create a variety of close relationships so as not to starve from lack of love and affection, I see why I regularly felt like a lonely, restless, boring, one-dimensional person in my marriage. While Evan certainly did appreciate many parts of me, there were some parts he could not comprehend. Since I didn't make time to build bonds with people who did understand, these vital, unrecognized pieces of my personality began dying a slow death inside me.

Contrary to myths and stories and popular belief, focusing on one person to fill your needs does not provide eternal protection against loneliness and isolation. In fact it's just the opposite. **Relying on one person for everything decreases your chances at human connection and increases your odds of feeling lonely and isolated.**

It's sort of like choosing spinach as your only vegetable at every meal. Eating tons of spinach may not be bad for you, but it is much better to pick a variety of vegetables, filling your bodywith the range of vitamins and nutrients it needs.

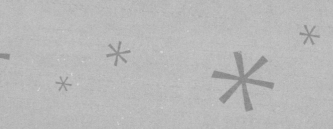

I recently began learning the Lindy Hop. This is a partner dance, and since I am single I attend a studio that doesn't require a person to be a part of a pair in order to join in the lessons. This open policy creates classes where couples mix together with unattached men and women, a formula certain to ferment interesting dynamics. We learn the dance by forming two concentric circles, one with leads and one with follows, and spend the entire period practicing footwork and perfecting technique while rotating from partner to partner around the circle so that each lead gets the opportunity to dance with each follow and vice versa. But not everybody rotates. Most often the couples in class choose to spend the entire hour dancing only with their significant other. We singles, however, are forced to rotate around the circle, forced to shake the sweaty hands of strangers, forced to get comfortable with a new partner every few minutes.

You might assume that the couples in class have it better than us singles. After all, they have an established rapport with their dance partners, sparing them the awkward, getting-to-know-you moments that we singles sometimes experience when dancing with an unfamiliar face for the first time. You would think that this comfort would allow the couples to be relaxed in their bodies, to move freely and thus become confident, stylish, accomplished dancers long before the rest of us. This is not what happens, though. What happens is that the singles learn quicker, becoming confident, stylish, accomplished dancers long before those couples who remain attached at the hip.

It's hard to say exactly why the singles become better dancers than the couples. Perhaps it's because the singles are on their best behavior, listening carefully to the instruction, moving attentively, exercising patience, working very hard not to look like idiots in front of people they've only just met. The couples, on the other hand, have a tendency to be overly casual about the whole process. They space out, they hold their arms sloppily, and when moves don't flow together as they should, the couples become easily frustrated. "I've seen couples yell at each other and leave in a huff," my Lindy Hop instructor told me. "That never happens with the people who rotate. It's sort of a basic law around here that if you want to keep your relationship intact *and* continue dancing, **you have to switch partners every once in awhile.**"

Of course, there are some couples who never experience these problems, but they are the exception, and so I cannot blame the couples who do repeat and perpetuate these adverse patterns. In fact, I can thoroughly relate to them, because before Evan and I were married we took swing dance lessons together. It did not go well.

We quit after three weeks.

The other reason I think couples in our classes don't learn to dance as well as the singles is that when a woman dances only with one partner she begins to overcompensate for his mistakes while he does the same for hers. Successful partner dancing requires a lead to communicate each move with decisive actions and a follow to listen intently with her body and respond fluidly to what she hears. The best way for dancers to fully understand their respective roles is by joining with different partners and feeling a variety of connections, movements, and styles. Couples who never separate don't really become good dancers so much as they become good at reading one particular person's body and method. These couples are not dancing, but are simply shifting about while making dissatisfying and unnecessary compromises.

That's what happened for Evan and me. When it came to swing dancing, Evan was a timid and vague lead, while I was an anxious and hasty follow. Evan barely lifted his arm and I turned; he stood still and I kept moving. Our teacher tried to instruct us. "You should be more assertive," she told Evan. "And you!" she said to me, "You need to stop back-leading." And so twice a week for three weeks Evan and I spent dance class scolding each other. Be more assertive! Stop back-leading! Now, looking back, I see that had we rotated partners, Evan and I would have been forced to work out our individual issues, because lord knows we are too polite to reprimand strangers. Perhaps Evan could have danced with a woman who stood still until he cued her. Perhaps I could have danced with a man who led firmly, forcing me to relinquish control.

I enjoy more success with dancing now that I am a single student, and for that I must thank the many partners who have moved me around the floor. Matt is energetic and unpredictable, James is subtle and smooth, Darren is playful and likes to invent new moves, Adam often gets off beat, but his smile and sense of humor make it no big deal, and Cole is so attentive, so sensual that when he puts his hand on my back and brings me close, I feel like I am the only woman in the entire world that matters to him. I must rely on different parts of my personality in order to dance with each of these guys, and I wouldn't trade any of them. I have grown so much.

If I were to dance with Evan again today, things would be different. At least on my part. **I would wait patiently until he felt ready to move.** I would remain attentive and present with him for the entire song. When we finished I would hug Evan and say, "Thank you," and then I would encourage him to dance with others. I would never again insist that we remain so tightly bound. I would never again force upon him my vision of how the dance should look.

Dancing is not something you do with your head. **It is something you feel with your body.** And while the mind can be helpful in the beginning stages of comprehension, ultimately dancing is best when thought has been abandoned. A woman learns to dance by dancing, by being completely present in the moment and allowing every cell in her body to bask in the pleasure of being spun around the floor and moved in a new way.

Dancing is best when you stop worrying, "How do I look? Am I doing this right? Do you think this guy likes dancing with me?" And so it is with love. **Love is best when you stop analyzing it and positioning it and trying to decipher its meaning.** Love is best when it flows freely and worst when it is conserved and given only to a select few. Your mother, your sister, the guy you just started dating, your boss, your barista, your annoying next door neighbor, your high school sweetheart, your best friend, the acquaintance you see from time to time, the solicitor who calls just as you sit down to dinner: you can be love to all of them.

six

**He Loves Me,
I Love Him Not.
I Love Him,
He Loves Me Not.**

One of the trickiest parts about being single is dealing with unrequited love. As single women it seems that we are either evading the advances of men we don't want or pining for the attention of men who don't want us.

I was endlessly flattered when the guy standing ahead of me in the coffee shop's line turned and remarked, "Great coat!" While I always welcome such praise, this particular compliment on that particular afternoon offered me the exact amount of validation that I desperately needed. I had recently broken up with the first man I had dated seriously since my divorce. I adored that man and our split hung heavily on my heart. It was winter and the coat I wore as I stood in line for a tall cappuccino was metallic red, very warm and, in my opinion, quite stylish. My ex-boyfriend, however, hated the coat and had no qualms about saying so. Since our split I thought a lot about my ex's disapproval of my funky fashion sense. While this was not the overt cause of our breakup, I couldn't help but wonder if the fate of our relationship would have been different had I dressed more conservatively.

I thanked my fellow coffee consumer for his compliment. "I appreciate it," I said. "I often worry that this coat is too much." The man shook his head, "No way. It's awesome." I sat down feeling lighter than I had in awhile. This man's generous remark seemed like a gift from the heavens, a reminder that **I did possess beauty and allure** and that men who appreciated my unique style did exist in this world.

Unfortunately my moment of existential relief was in fact just a moment. I sat at my table reading the newspaper for only a few minutes before the man from line walked over and handed me his business card. "I'd like to get together with you sometime," he said. **My heart fell.** While I was truly grateful for his earlier compliment, I wasn't interested in dating him or anybody else for that matter. My psyche was still bruised and tender from my breakup. Besides, I do not believe in romantic rebounding, and even if I did I could tell that this man, although kind and sweet for sure, was not a right match for me.

As I opened my mouth to graciously decline his offer, the man cut me off. "I don't have time to talk right now," he said. "I'm in a hurry so, you know, just call me." Then he rushed out the door, leaving me slightly confused and incredibly annoyed. "How rude!" I thought. "If a man wants to date a woman he should not do so by tossing her a business card. He should ask properly and stand by while she responds. **What a coward! What a jerk!**" And so it was that my heavenly gift brought with it a worldly burden.

The business card remained in my wallet while I viscerally felt the man's nervous energy awaiting my call. I agonized and vacillated over my next step. What was I to do? A meeting was out of the question, for I learned long ago that dates arranged out of pity and obligation spin tangled webs, the undoing of which always resulting in terribly hurt feelings for at least one of the parties involved. But to ignore his offer completely seemed insensitive and cruel. While the man had certainly behaved in a socially awkward manner, I could tell from their encounter that he wasn't a sleaze with ill intentions. I understood that he was sensitive and knew that turning him down would require white gloves. The more I thought about it, the more annoyed I became until I eventually worked myself into a furious mess. I became livid at the man for cornering me like this. My heart and mind were already filled with enough worries. The last thing I needed to think about were the feelings of a complete stranger.

The situation remained this way for three solid days until an unexpected wave of wisdom rose inside me one evening as I sat at my computer, half working to complete a pressing deadline and half brooding about the man from coffee. The wave started by gently lapping at my heart, but rapidly grew to a strong groundswell that engulfed all my feelings, worries, and ideas. This surge did not sing sounds of the ocean, but instead spoke straight advice. **"Be honest. Be humble. Be kind.** And remember: You have been in this situation before." This was the voice of my subconscious breaking past my ego and finally gaining the attention of my conscious ear.

Everyone has a connection to the divine. All people have access to truth. Each of us has an untainted place inside that is innocent, pure, open, good. When we listen to the voice that speaks from this place, we feel relief. We feel light. We feel peace. When our actions are motivated from this sacred space, we cannot fail. We have no choice but to do the right thing.

So of course the words from my wave of wisdom were right on. I *had* been in this situation before. Only that time, the roles were reversed. It was I who handed my phone number to a man I just met at a coffee shop. He was the barista and I had felt a magnetic connection as I ordered my drink, a connection I didn't normally experience in casual encounters. But apparently this spark was one-sided, because when I wrote my phone number on a small napkin and passed it across the counter, the barista's buoyant smile sunk hard and fast. "Oh. Um. I'm sorry. I. Um. I'm dating somebody," he said. I knew the barista was lying.

When my subconscious reminded me of this incident that had occurred years before, my annoyance transformed to empathy. I remembered how quickly I fell smitten for that barista, and I understood how the man from the coffee shop line could have easily misinterpreted my thankful smile as an invitation to romance.

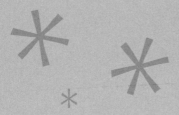

The next morning I removed the business card from my wallet and dialed the number on it. Secretly I prayed to get his voicemail, but the man himself answered the phone, providing me with a true test of my kindness and bravery. I told him in the most concise way I could that I was flattered by his interest, but that I was still pining for my ex, that my heart was raw, and that I was not yet open to exploring new relationships with men. I also thanked him again for his comment about my coat. I told him how my ex had hated that coat and how the compliment helped lift me from the dark place where I had been residing since our breakup. Finally I told the man that I hoped my inability to get together did not prevent him from reaching out to others in the future. The man listened quietly before responding, **"This is the most honest rejection I have ever received. Thank you."** And with that we wished each other good luck and said good-bye.

In the end I think I handled the situation just right. And so did the man. He remained tender and open and listened patiently even as I was turning him down. Isn't it wonderful when two people treat each other gently even though they disagree, show compassion even when their desires diverge?

One of the hardest parts about being single is keeping your heart open. It seems we are always hearing no, always saying no. We are either rejecting or getting rejecting. Connections fall flat, hopes die, affections go unreciprocated, expectations are rarely met. **It's no wonder we build walls around our hearts.** It's no wonder we feel disillusioned. It's no wonder we become cynics. It is very hard to live yes and no simultaneously.

Loretta has been let down by love. She loved a man who wouldn't be faithful and another with a critical tongue. She loved a man who said he didn't want children only to break up with her and find himself a new woman with whom he promptly—and happily—produced a bouncing baby boy. Eventually Loretta loved a man with the kindest soul she had ever encountered. They dated for two years and Loretta was certain she would become his wife. In the end, however, for reasons Loretta cannot quite articulate, the two took separate paths.

Since then Loretta has had an ample serving of less than tasteful men. More than anything, Loretta longs to click with a man in that easy, I-feel-like-I've-known-you-my-whole-life kind of way. This connection is not happening organically, however, so Loretta recently decided to take charge of the situation and sign up for an online dating service. Within one week Loretta had her first date arranged. **She was excited, but that excitement turned to disappointment** when she arrived at the restaurant only to discover that the man had blatantly lied about his height and quite possibly used Photoshop to enhance the snapshot that accompanied his profile.

The night quickly progressed from bad to worse. Loretta had not even finished her first martini when her date announced, "I don't usually go out with women your age. You're all bitter and dying to have babies. It drives me nuts." Loretta couldn't believe her ears. She wanted to throw her drink in his face. She wanted to scream. She was in her mid-thirties. He was nearly fifty. Where did this man get the nerve to make such a statement? But instead of making a scene, Loretta did something else that she had never before done on a date: **she walked out.**

The man's nasty words lingered, popping into her mind unexpectedly while grocery shopping or washing her hair. It made Loretta bristle. She wished terrible things upon him. She wished all his teeth would fall out and that he would go to the dentist only to have his new teeth fall out again the next day. She wished he would spend his whole life in the dentist chair. Loretta hated that man. "He's a clueless ego maniac asshole loser," her inner voice yelled. Things continued this way for weeks until one night, while driving home from work after a day of particularly grueling meetings, Loretta thought about his comment once again. This time instead of raging, she sobbed. The tears bombarded her eyes so fiercely that Loretta had to pull over to the side of the road where she sat, a blubbering mess, for forty minutes.

At the end of her tearful episode, Loretta realized that although her date was out of line, and although she did not feel guilty for walking out on him that night, he had been right about one thing: she was bitter. She had allowed all her past hurts to pile up and build an impenetrable fortress around her heart. "I was skeptical of all men," she said. "I didn't want to be let down again, so I never let myself get excited about things like a man unexpectedly flirting or my friends wanting to set me up. I wasn't excited even if I was truly interested in the guy." The thing Loretta discovered as she thought about it more was that she always felt bad when a date went poorly whether she had high hopes or not. "I've decided it's better to be let down with an open heart than a closed heart, because at least with an open heart I know I've given it a shot."

Loretta's advice?
Make peace with the hurts
of your past without
projecting those hurts on
the men of your present.

You may think that holding back your expectations for love and remaining skeptical about the number of quality, relationship-worthy men in this world will spare you uncomfortable anguish. Such an attitude, however, is not protection, but poison. It will harden your heart, sour your perspective, diminish your spirit, and turn you into a person who is not very much fun to be around.

No matter how many times you have failed to find the kind of love you crave, know that it does exist for you. Believe that love lies just around the corner. Wait enthusiastically for it. Be an optimist. Let your hopes soar.

The bad news is that **you will experience many broken hearts living open and exposed in this way.** You will experience more broken hearts than the average person, which is actually a very wonderful, lucky thing. Who wants to be average anyway? Who wants to live in the same old, status quo, middle-of-the-road way? We must not aim for typical, but aim for exceptional, for miraculous, for divine.

The good news is that a broken
heart is a sign that you are alive,
that you are hopeful, that you
are giving love. A broken heart
need not kill you. A broken heart
need not deaden your soul.
A broken heart is healable,
but not preventable.

Many times I have felt the blinding, choking, nauseating pain that consumes the body when a heart is ripped in two. My heart broke when Evan and I first said aloud that our marriage was not working, when my ex-boyfriend mentioned casually over Chinese food that he hated my metallic red coat, when Colin Darington pretended to sprain his ankle as an excuse not to dance with me at our first junior high dance, when my coworker told me last week, in so many words, that she doesn't think I am particularly pretty, when editors at newspapers, magazines, online journals, and book publishers reject my work yet again. The list goes on and on and on and on and on. I'm sure you have a list like this as well. **There are too many broken hearts to remember, too many to count.**

So how are we to make peace with these hurts, so that they do not make us bitter and sabotage our chances at prosperity in the future? I have a psychologist friend who advises, **"Grieve. Grieve. Grieve. And when the grieving is done, move your energy."** She means sit in a bathtub filled with warm, sweet-scented water and sob. She means take a long nap in the middle of the day. She means don't force a smile if you aren't in the mood. She also means that the minute the heavy ache of sadness lifts, you must do something to infuse your being with fresh energy. Take a walk, join an art class, throw a party. You grieve so you **don't repress your sadness,** and you move your energy so you don't remain stuck.

When it comes to dating and romance, unrequited love and broken hearts, how long you have known somebody is inconsequential. **It is always painful when love does not flourish as hoped,** when opportunity leads to a dead end. Sometimes a first date falling flat brings up more sadness than the end of a relationship that lasted for years.

And so we must address all our disappointments, big and small. As my friend Loretta has learned, "If you don't deal with your upset and anger it will accumulate. It will bury your lovely, loving, playful womanly spirit. We need that spirit. We need it thriving. Nothing else really matters if your spirit is dead. **A lively spirit, that's what makes life worth living."**

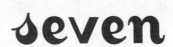

seven

**Every Day She Did
the Impossible**

There is always a chance to learn something new, to break deadening routines, to calm anxiety, to heal sorrow, to experience love. These opportunities exist as long as you want them to. Life is not over until you decide it is.

I was raised by a single mother. She could tell you a lot about heartache, a lot about mind-numbing loneliness. She could tell you about humiliation and desperation. She could tell you about wanting, about wishing, about longing for everything to be different. She could tell you about unanswered prayers. But my mom could also tell you a lot about **optimism and hard work and success against all odds.** She could tell you about creativity, about heart-exploding gratitude, about witnessing magnificence in the mundane. My mom could tell you about miracles. She could tell you about joy.

When my mom was twenty-three she married her college sweetheart. When my mom was twenty-nine, her handsome, dependable, picture-perfect husband died unexpectedly of a heart attack. When my mom was thirty-one she met the man who would become my father and married him more out of loneliness than love. Two years later, he ran off with another woman and most of my mom's money. And so there she was, standing alone in a big suburban house, a thirty-five-year-old divorced widow with a newborn baby girl and mortgage payments through the roof.

Even before she was a teenager my mother dreamt of having a husband. More than anything else in this world she wanted to build a life with a man. World travel, education, career advancement, romantic flings—these things did not interest her in the way commitment, stability, and companionship did. When I was four years old my mom met a man who she says took her breath away. His name was Ashoka, and on their first date, while they perused the shelves of a small bookshop, as my mom reached for a thin paperback, he laid his hand on top of hers. In that single touch Ashoka offered my **mom more compassion and tenderness then she had ever experienced.** The problem? He was a gypsy, a headstrong intellectual, a spiritual seeker uninterested in settling down in the suburbs with a woman and a child.

I won't get into all the details of their long relationship, but I will tell you this: Ten years after their first meeting, Ashoka got sick and was diagnosed with an aggressive, terminal cancer. And thus my mom found herself once again in the middle of an unbearable, heart-wrenching situation with a man. I imagine my mom must have been so angry. I imagine she must have wondered what she had done to deserve such struggle. I imagine she must have felt guilty, like a failure, like she was being punished. I imagine she must have felt sorry for herself. I imagine she must have felt anguish and excruciating isolation. I imagine my mom must have felt a million emotions all at once.

Whatever emotions my mom may have felt, she did not have the luxury to entertain them for long. She had a teenage girl in her house and a dying man in her bed. Looking back on it now that I am older, now that I too am a woman, I am amazed how my mom found strength to work full time, to wash laundry, to arrange for hospice care, and still prepare a brown-bag lunch for me to take to school with a little note inside that read, "I love you." I know that every day women all around the world summon staggering amounts of strength to perform duties like these and some even harder. When I think of my mother and all of these those women, **I am amazed. I am humbled and I am amazed.**

When Ashoka died, he left my mom a little bit of money and a book on papier-mâché. My mom first became interested in this art form before Ashoka got sick, when the two of them strolled into an artsy furniture store and saw a huge papier-mâché bowl sitting on a pedestal near the front door. My mom fell in love with the bowl. Ashoka said he'd buy it for her, but at $300, my mom wouldn't allow it. Ashoka insisted. My mom resisted. "You're not spending your money on that," she said. "Besides, I could probably make that. I'll learn papier-mâché and make one for myself." They left the store without the bowl, and it wasn't until after Ashoka died, with his final gift as her inspiration, that my mother first attempted papier-mâché.

It has taken my mom thirteen years and countless pounds of newsprint and paste to perfect her papier-mâché technique. She finally has it down. My mom makes whimsical bracelets and bowls covered with hand-painted flowers, photocopies of vintage doilies from her gigantic collection, and any other paper that catches her eye. Last December my mother displayed her creations at a local gallery where she sold twelve of her bracelets and one of her beautiful black-and-white bowls. Just think of it, my mom has had so many titles. She has been a daughter, a wife, a widow, a graduate student, a social worker, a divorcée, a single mother, a public speaker, a caretaker, and now, at the sweet age of sixty-two, **my dear mother is an artist.**

0On the inside of some of my mom's handmade bracelets you will find the sentence, **"Every day she did the impossible."** I love this. It seems that so many of us, so much of the time, are asked by the world to do things that feel utterly impossible. And so many of us, so much of the time, find strength from God knows where to simply do that utterly impossible.

One of the greatest resources we have in this world is the wisdom of the women who have gone before us. As young women we know next to nothing. We are just babies. We are only starting out. **Let us not be righteous in our youth, but respectful.** Let us seek inspiration from older generations. Let us listen instead of speak, let us admire their beauty instead of flaunt our own. Let us be modest and full of reverence, for if we are lucky we will be sixty someday too. And eighty. And maybe even one hundred.

When you find yourself angry and lonely and hopeless in your single life, don't seek advice only from your peers and from pop culture. Find an older woman whom you admire, a woman wise from experience, and ask her for guidance. Find out what her pains have been and how she has dealt with those pains. **As she shares with you the stories of her life, listen intently, and take her words to heart.**

Last week I met a new acquaintance for happy hour cocktails after work. As we sat sipping our gin and tonics and munching on crispy tempura prawns, my new acquaintance told me that she would like to have Botox injections in her forehead. Botox and she is twenty-eight. Twenty-eight with smooth skin, twenty-eight with wrinkles visible only under a magnifying glass and extremely bright lights. She also told me that she wants her tummy tucked, her thighs lipo-sucked, and a small amount of loose skin removed from the back of her arms. "I'd get it all!" she exclaimed. Twenty-eight and she'd get it all.

There is a woman who comes into the gym where I work. She is much older than twenty-eight, she has not had Botox, and she is beautiful. Her hair is silver and she wears it in a smooth, sleek bob that falls just below her chin. Lines surround her eyes and lips, and her skin is slightly freckled from all those years in the sun. Four days each week she walks on the treadmill, then rides the bike, then stretches in the small room downstairs. I love to look at her. **She is strong. She is confident.** She is joyful. She possesses the type of beauty that cannot be created in a surgeon's office, beauty that is not threatened by twenty-eight year olds.

I hope to grow old like the woman at the gym and not like my new acquaintance. I don't want to spend forever hiding behind hair dye. I don't want injections that annihilate my expressions. I don't want to undergo surgery for vanity's sake. I do not want to harbor a perverse obsession with youth, a ridiculous, arbitrary idea of perfection. As I grow I want to embrace my age, to trust that my beauty will deepen, not disappear. I want to be strong. I want to value wisdom. I want to welcome joy.

I want to embrace everything that life offers me. I want to take comfort in the wild, mysterious natural order of things. I don't want to spend my life watching the clock. I don't want to punch a time card. I don't want to make a checklist. I don't want to live my life like a day planner, scheduling and organizing. I do not want to panic, "When am I going to meet Mr. Right? When am I going to have babies? When am I going to get a book published? When am I going to see my first gray hair? When am I going to be a success? When am I going to die?" I want to wait for the events of my life the way a little girl waits for Santa Claus, excited, wide-eyed, wonderful. **I want to applaud each item that fills the stocking of my life.** I want to live like this all the way through my last breath.

I have a photograph of my mother when she was eight years old. In it she wears a dress and shiny black leather shoes and stands on the sidewalk in front of the house where she grew up. She poses with one hand on her hip, her lips puckered to kiss the air. Her eyes are vibrant and assured as if to say, **"Come on world! I'm ready for you! Grab my hand! Let's run! Let's go!"**

I have another photograph of my mom taken just last summer. In it she is as sweet, as innocent, as juicy as she was in that picture taken more than fifty years ago. She looks straight into the camera and smiles, and you can see immediately that my mother has not let the disappointments of her life diminish her spirit. On many occasions heartache has come to her, but **heartache has not overcome her, it has not become her.**

This is how we must live.
We must be strong. We must be
grateful. We must be kind. We
must be humble. We must be
centered. We must be patient. We
must be awake. Remember: Being
a single woman is not easy, but it
is not the kiss of death either.

Oh, Wild Woe! I know you have not had your last visit with my heart, therefore come as you will. I will sob with you over tea until all my tears have dried and then I will ask you to leave because I have other company I would like to entertain.. And if you will not go, persistent Woe, I will mix you with my secret marinara sauce. I will simmer you with basil and oregano and serve you over al dente linguine. I will papier-mâché you onto bracelets and bowls. I will take you to my acting class and force you to help me perform a moving monologue. I will twirl with you on the dance floor. I will strap you to my back and ride my bicycle past the city and into the country. I will ride with you through the sunset, into darkness, until the stars and moon touch us with their light. I will ride until your sorrowful howls turn to giggles of joy.

The purpose of this life is not to find one perfect, all-encompassing mate. It is not to mindlessly have babies. It is not to gain notoriety or fame or fortune. The purpose of this life is to find that place inside yourself where you can remain peaceful and optimistic no matter what the outside world throws your way.

Oh, sweet God, I cannot get my mind around you. I cannot comprehend this bizarre, lonely world. I cannot understand the universe or the planets or why it is that some people suffer so much pain while others float through life on soft clouds. I cannot predict my future nor can I undo the mistakes of my past. All I can do is let go. All I can do is throw my arms open and exclaim, "Come to me!" **Kiss me, Life!** Kiss me, Divine Uncertainty! Kiss me, Gorgeous Man! Kiss me! I am ready! I am worthy! I am single! I am excited! I am beautiful! I am alive!

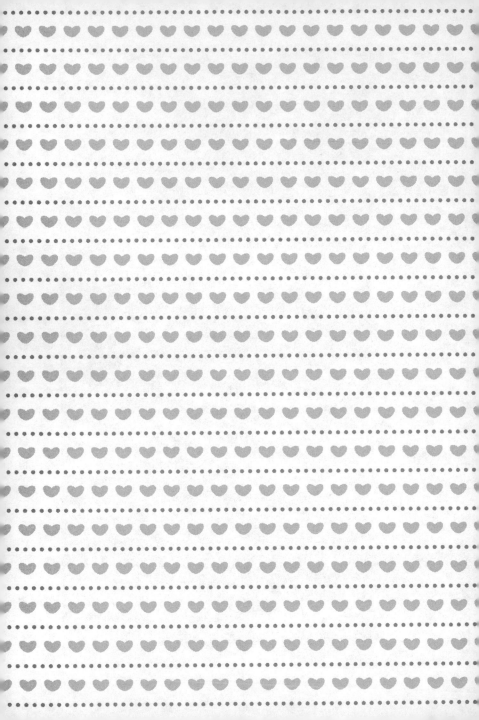

About the Author

Amanda Ford began her writing career at age 6, when her mother gave her a journal filled with pink pages to record her daily adventures. Today, at the age of twenty-seven, Amanda has authored three books, including *Be True to Yourself*, *Retail Therapy*, and *Between Mother and Daughter*, which she co-authored with her mother, Judy. Amanda's work has been featured in publications such as *Real Simple*, *Glamour*, *Good Housekeeping*, *Redbook*, *The Seattle Times*, and *The Chicago Tribune*. When she isn't scribbling in her journal or typing wildly at her computer, you can find Amanda blazing trails on her mountain bike, ballroom dancing, or sipping tea with her grandmother. She lives in Seattle, in a tiny apartment by a lake. You can reach Amanda through her website *www.oholive.com*.

Acknowledgments

It is amazing that this book, being so diminutive in size, required the input, the support, the hard work of so many people.

Thank you first to Judy "Lily D" Ford. Without your persistence and your insistence this book would have never made it off my laptop. Thank you to Brenda Knight for always being on my team. Thank you to Jan Johnson, Michael Kerber, Donna Linden, Bonni Hamilton, Skye Wentworth, Pam Suwinsky, Jessie Dacher, Caroline Pincus, Jordan Overby, and the many "unseen hands" at Red Wheel/Weiser for working tirelessly on my behalf. The book exceeds my hopes. Thank you.

Thank you to my sweet ex-husband for allowing me to share our story. And thank you to the handsome men who have driven me to distraction over the years. Here's to homegrown spinach, midnight bicycle rides, living room blues dances, awkward text messages, shocking love notes, innumerable attempts at sushi and even more cocktails. Thank you for the tenderness and the heartache. I adore you all to pieces.

Thank you to Karen Salmansohn, Bella DePaulo, Diane Mapes, and Sasha Cagen for your generous words of support. And thank you to everyone whose story is shared in these pages so that others might feel less alone.

And of course, thank you to my amazing family of lifelong friends who keep me sane and always support me more than they should. Alexander "Rikki Rikki" Lieu, Melanie O'Dell, Phillip "Shiny" Johnson, Sarah Smith White, Adrienne Schaefer, Becky Masters, Gethen Bassett, Jean Theisen, Kathy "Jean Bean" Sorensen, Phyllis "Grandma" Sorensen. You inspire me endlessly. One million hugs and kisses to you all.

To Our Readers

Conari Press, an imprint of Red Wheel/Weiser, publishes books on topics ranging from spirituality, personal growth, and relationships to women's issues, parenting, and social issues. Our mission is to publish quality books that will make a difference in people's lives—how we feel about ourselves and how we relate to one another. We value integrity, compassion, and receptivity, both in the books we publish and in the way we do business.

Our readers are our most important resource, and we value your input, suggestions, and ideas about what you would like to see published. Please feel free to contact us, to request our latest book catalog, or to be added to our mailing list.

Conari Press

An imprint of Red Wheel/Weiser, LLC

500 Third Street, Suite 230

San Francisco, CA 94107

www.redwheelweiser.com